Natural Remedies for Menopause

A Complete List of Herbs and Vitamins for Natural Menopause Relief

by Betsy Sanders

Table of Contents

Introduction

So, you've approached the age of menopause, and are starting to undergo its effects. While contemporary medicine has so far used Hormone Replacement Therapy in order to manage the symptoms of menopause, recent studies have conclusively shown that HRT is linked to an increased risk of stroke, blood clots, cardiac disease, and cancer.

In light of these side-effects that pose a severe health hazard to HRT patients, an increasing number of women are turning to alternative and natural remedies in order to manage their discomfort in this phase of their lives.

But, with the overwhelming and sometimes contrary information available on the internet, how does one differentiate the helpful sources from the harmful ones? How does one gain a comprehensive knowledge of the products and therapies that genuinely seem to help, versus the ones that are often touted but rarely work? While everyone talks about Black Cohosh as a good natural remedy, why are doctors strongly advising against its use in women? The answers to all these questions and more are found within this book guide.

Are you ready to get rid of the uncomfortable hot flashes? Are you ready to improve your quality of life and your physical well-being by managing the inconveniences of this phase in your life? And are you ready to do all of this in a *natural* and healthy way? Let's get started!

Chapter 1: Let's Talk Menopause

Menopause is a normal progression in a woman's life, and essentially marks the permanent end of her menstrual periods. Its onset can begin as a completely normal phase, or can be caused by external factors such as surgery, radiation, or chemotherapy.

"Menopausal transition" or "Peri-menopause" is a term used for the period of time before and after the last period ever, while a woman's hormonal levels are still fluctuating severely. It consists of three stages:

"Pre-menopause" is used to denote the span of time before the last period, when the symptoms begin and persist while a woman is still experiencing her menses.

"Natural menopause" is considered to have been completed in a woman when she has not had a menses for 12 consecutive months.

"Post-menopause" is used to denote the term of a woman's natural life which occurs after the date of menopause. So, if a woman has had no menstrual flow at all for a full two years, she is considered to be two years into post-menopause.

Due to the complications of aging, there are several symptoms which, though attributed to menopause, may be more strongly related to aging itself. However, studies have at least enabled us to garner evidence to prove that menopause has the strongest links with the following of those symptoms:

- Hot flashes and night sweats (rarely, cold flashes)

- Vaginal dryness, itchiness, loss of elasticity

- Reasoning, concentration, and memory problems

- Physical discomfort – exhaustion, stiff or painful joints, muscle and back pain

- Mood swings – depression, anxiety, irritability

- Some women complain of urinary incontinence after menopause

- Possible risk of atherosclerosis

- Migraines

- Urinary urgency

- Increasingly prone to vaginal inflammation and infection

- Watery vaginal discharge

- Breast atrophy and/or tenderness

- Osteopenia and increased risk of Osteoporosis

- Formication: Itchy burning, pins and needles, a sensation reminiscent to ants crawling over the skin

- Dry and decreasingly elastic skin

- Disturbance in sleep patterns, or even insomnia

- Decreased libido

As I mentioned before, contemporary medicine had been using Hormone Replacement Therapy in order to mitigate the various symptoms of menopause, until recent studies showed that HRT patients were at an increased risk for heart disease, blood clots, stroke, and breast cancer. While the risks differed, this applied to both combination as well as estrogen-only HRT. Further studies showed that even after discontinuing HRT usage, the former patients remained at increased risk for cancer, clots and stroke, even though the risks for heart disease diminished.

This precipitated a global movement where women eschewed the contemporary treatments in favor of natural remedies. However, it's important to differentiate between "natural" and "safe" as one doesn't necessarily mean the other. Several scientific studies into the effects of many touted natural remedies have delivered inconclusive results, with very few of them showing definite improvement in the quality of life of menopausal women. Thus, we've tried our best to deliver a comprehensive store of knowledge here, with popular remedies listed along with the current opinion of scientific study on their effectiveness. However, before we launch into the list, it is of vital importance to mention one point.

Before using any alternative or natural remedies that involve consumption of substances, inform and consult with your health-care practitioner to avoid any interactions with medicine which you may currently be prescribed or any other adverse affects due to your specific health condition. Also, it's far more effective to create a holistic and integrated health-care regimen in conjunction with the knowledge and experience of your doctor, than experiment with natural pharmacological substances on your own.

Chapter 2: Vitamins and Supplements for Menopause

Vitamin E – When applied to the vagina in topical oil form, it helps to improve lubrication. Vitamin E, consumed orally in a recommended dosage of 800 mg a day, can help relieve night sweats and hot flashes as well as manage mood swings.

Vitamin D – With age, the ability of women's bodies to absorb vitamin D decreases, increasing their risk for bone density loss, which makes this supplement crucial for consumption. This vitamin serves as an essential building block in a body, and is responsible for bone renewal, normal cell growth, and hormonal balance.

Calcium – Since increased risk of osteoporosis is one of the bigger results of menopause, it becomes essential to consume about 1,500 to 2,000 mg of calcium in order to promote healthy bone density.

DHEA – This is a naturally occurring substance in the human body, the levels of which decrease with age. DHEA is synthesized and sold as a dietary supplement and is believed to show some benefits with regards to hot flashes and decreased libido.

However, it must be noted that hard scientific evidence has yet to support this notion with clear proof.

Vitamin B complex – This is a really effective dietary supplement, especially for women wishing to relieve menopausal symptoms. It promotes healthy mucous membranes, including those of the vagina. It acts as an antioxidant, helps alleviate memory loss, improves concentration, manages depression and mood swings. It helps in correcting loss of appetite, helps in keeping skin, nails and hair healthy. It also helps reduce anxiety and fatigue, and promotes good sleep. It can also reduce blood cholesterol, dilate blood vessels and help in relief from menopausal migraines.

Glucosamine supplements – Available readily as dietary supplements, Glucosamine helps produce more collagen and helps control the enzymes which break down cartilage. This is invaluable as a remedy against joint problems and arthritis issues which are brought on by menopause

Chapter 3: Herbs, Foods, and Other Natural Remedies for Menopause

<u>Black Cohosh</u> (Cimicifuga racemosa) – This is one of the most widely-used and espoused natural remedies to relieve hot flashes, help manage depression, and vaginal atrophy. However, U.S pharmacopeia experts suggest that women should consult their health-care practitioners without fail before its use, since it has been linked to liver problems, abdominal pains, and jaundice.

<u>Red Clover</u> – Like the last discussed herb, this remedy is believed to have greatly beneficial properties because it contains phyto-estrogens (plant estrogens). These phyto-estrogens are believed to mimic the properties of estrogen in the human body, and help prevent osteoporosis and reduce bone resorption. However, research studies in the U.S. suggest that there may be some link between phyto-estrogen and hormone-sensitive tissue like mammary tissue, and so may be linked with breast cancer. Doctors caution that women who are at an increased risk for hormone-related diseases or health conditions should be especially careful while using red clover.

<u>Wild Yam</u> – This natural plant is widely touted to help relieve menopausal symptoms, and is often marketed as such. It contains diosgenin, which is used to create a synthetic version of progesterone in labs, and may also contain some chemicals that weakly resemble estrogen. However, studies have recently proved without doubt that wild yam is conclusively useless in management of menopausal symptoms. The chemical diosgenin, which is used as the basis of its marketing, cannot be naturally converted to progesterone in the body, and needs a lengthy process in a lab to be converted to that chemical compound.

St. John's Wort – Another popular herb used in the United States, St. John's wort has been used as an alternative treatment for menopausal mood swings, better sleep, relaxation, and management of depression and anxiety. Derived from Hypericum perforatum, a wild flowering plant, the leaves and flowers are dried after being harvested. It can be brewed as a tea, or be consumed orally as a pill or a liquid. It is important to note that while this herb is effective in cases of mild depression, it shows no remarkable benefit in severe cases.

Ginseng – Used for over five millennia by the Chinese for its health benefits, Ginseng is effective as treatment to manage fatigue, stress, and anxiety. It is also beneficial for improving sleep patterns and helps improve one's overall sense of well-being. Ginseng can be consumed by brewing it in a tea, or consuming it as a powder or herbal extract to be added to juices or shakes.

Soy – This is held to be extremely beneficial to one's overall health, and may be effective in reducing menopausal symptoms. Soy contains isoflavones, which are also phyto-estrogens, and besides other phyto-estrogenic benefits may also lower cholesterol. However, it is officially recommended to consume soy in food forms, and not as a tablet or powder.

Flaxseeds – These are a source of phyto-estrogens as well, and are held to be extremely effective in managing menopausal symptoms. These can be ground and added to cereal or yogurt for easy consumption.

Natural Salves – Calendula and Comfrey – These natural salves can be purchased, and are believed to be particularly helpful for vaginal dryness. They have healing and anti-microbial properties as well that help fight the increased vulnerability to vaginal infections. Also, Comfrey contains a natural constituent compound called allantoin which promotes regeneration of healthy skin tissue. These salves can be used once or twice every day, as needed.

Sage (Salvia officinalis) – The use of sage as an aid to reduce sweating and night flashes was popular for a very long time. Recently, research has backed up that anecdotal knowledge with scientific evidence. The studies showed that consumption of a single sage tablet every day reduced hot flashes by half within 4 weeks, and showed continued improvement in that area further on as well. In fact, the women who had the most severe hot flashes reported 80 to 100% decrease in hot flashes, and the ones who still had them from time to time reported a marked decrease in their severity.

If you're unable to get the sage tablet, this herb works just as effectively when brewed as tea. You can even add agave nectar, honey, or lemon to the hot or iced sage tea to make it feel far more refreshing.

Maca (Lepidium meyenii) – Maca is an herb that originates from the Andes Mountains in Peru, and has several beneficial properties for women suffering from menopausal symptoms. This is a non-estrogenic herb, which means that it does not contain any estrogen. Instead, this class of herbs works on stimulating the hormone centers in the human body, and promote the body to produce its own hormones more effectively so that it doesn't need any external aid in regulating its internal environment. The bio-active alkaloids in Maca nourish and stimulate the glands in the body, and so help in correcting the body's hormonal balance.

If you cannot get access to the herb through convenient means, it is also available in the form of supplementary pills such as Macafem.

Chasteberry (Vitex Agnus castus) – The berries of the Agnus castus plant have long been used for treating the symptoms of PMS while in the peri-menopause phase, when the hormonal levels in the body are still fluctuating wildly. However, caution must be exercised that the herb is not consumed at the same time as other prescription hormonal medicines.

Valerian Root (Valeriana officinalis) – The root of the valerian plant is an effective medicine for stress and anxiety. It works well as a relaxant and a sleep aid, and so is an invaluable natural remedy for women suffering from sleep-related problems brought on by menopause. It can be used as a powdered form of the root, or as pre-prepared pills and other such supplements for consumption.

Devil's Claw (Harpagophytum procumbens) – For those who've found Arnica as an insufficiently effective remedy against pain, the root of the Devil's

Claw is widely used as a treatment for painful joints and aching muscles. It is available in tablet form for convenient consumption.

Gingko (Gingko biloba) – This is one of the most researched medicines from those which have long been used as natural remedies in Chinese culture. Gingko helps regulate normal blood circulation, and has been shown to be especially effective in promoting better circulation to the brain. This is particularly useful for dealing with the memory and concentration problems associated with menopause.

Millet – This is useful as a good source of silicon – an essential element helpful in trace amounts during consumption in order to improve the strength and structure of hair. It is also well-known for its protein quality, which provides keratin and is useful in keeping hair, skin, and nails healthier.

Dong Quai (Angelica sinensis) – Dong Quai is notable as an effective medicinal herb to be used for relief against menopausal symptoms, particularly since it isn't an estrogenic herb. It is well known for its ability to maintain and support the normal hormonal balance in women. It is important to mention that this herb should not be consumed by women who are experiencing heavy bleeding.

Evening Primrose (Oenethera biennis) – Women suffering from menopausal symptoms often experience hair loss, eczema, dry skin, and tender breasts, as well as longer healing times due to lower estrogen levels. Topical administration of Evening primrose oil helps moderate these symptoms since it contains gamma-linolenic acid (GLA) which is an essential fatty acid that helps promote better prostaglandin synthesis. Black currant oil is another natural remedy that works in a similar fashion.

Red Raspberry – The leaves of the red raspberry plant are extremely nutritious – containing vitamins E, G, C, B and A as well as Calcium, Phosphorus, Niacin, Iron and Manganese - and have helpful therapeutic uses for women suffering from menopausal symptoms. This herb helps in maintaining healthy nails, skin, bones and teeth, in maintaining the balance of hormonal levels in women, reduces excessive menstruation and spasms in the uterus and intestines, helps in replenishing iron content in blood and works as an effective treatment for dysentery and diarrhea as well as a great mouthwash for sores and infected gums.

Mistletoe – When consumed as a tea, Mistletoe is an extremely effective remedy to regulate blood pressure and counter dizziness, heart flutters, excessive menstruation, anxiety and hot flushes. It also works as a great energizer. Mistletoe nourishes and benefits the glandular system, helps improve metabolism, nurtures the pancreas, and so is regarded with great favor among the myriad of herbal medicines used for relief from menopausal symptoms.

Motherwort – This herb is an extremely potent neurotonic and cardiotonic (nourishes the nervous system and heart). It works well as a relaxant and is effective in reducing anxiety and hot flashes, especially if they lead to tachycardia (rapid heartbeat).

Seaweed – Long known for possessing several therapeutic and nourishing properties, seaweed can be consumed regularly and helps in regulating and healing various negative conditions associated with menopause and others associated with aging in women as well – osteoporosis, mastitis, fibroids, ovarian cysts, cancer (breast/uterine/ovarian), fibro-cystic breast distress, infertility, water retention, hot flashes, fatigue, lack of lubrication, loss of calcium, mood swings, irregularity in menstrual cycles, etc.

Hawthorn (Crataegus laevigata) - This is a particularly useful cardio-regulating medicine which helps dilate coronary arteries, provides more blood to the muscles of the heart, reduces risk of heart attack, corrects low blood pressure, and is particularly effective in controlling heart palpitations if someone experiences fluttering or racing of the heart, and helps prevent cardiac arrhythmia.

Garlic (**Allium sativum**) - This well-known household ingredient not only lowers blood pressure but glucose, lipid, and cholesterol levels as well. It also has antibiotic and antifungal actions, prevents the formation of blood clots, strengthens the immune system and helps to protect the liver.

Hops – This popular ingredient used in brewing beer has been known to hold sedative, hypnotic, and therapeutic properties since ancient times. Research shows that extract from hops has estrogenic activity, and at a much stronger level than other phytoestrogenic plants. Studies have conclusively proven that hops provide that rare combination of medicinal efficacy and safety that is the ideal benchmark for a natural remedy.

Fish – While it is well known that fish meat is invaluable for its health benefits, the Omega-3 fatty acids are not only heart and cholesterol-friendly, but help in regulating mood swings as well.

Kava (**Piper methysticum**) – Although it is touted to help provide relief from hot flashes, there is no scientific evidence supporting this claim. However, it has shown to be effective in reducing anxiety and so is helpful with managing such mood problems which are caused by menopause. But it must be mentioned that Kava has been strongly linked to liver disease, and as a result is banned for distribution by various countries.

Milk Thistle – Used as a cleansing herb, especially by women going through menopause, milk thistle has several important therapeutic properties: it is liver protecting and cleansing, a natural antidepressant and mood stabilizer, it is preventative for storage of fat, it improves bile production and thus reduces constipation and liver damage or related problems, and it helps the body break down hormonal supplements.

Chamomile – It is a well-known traditional remedy for anxiety and stress, indigestion and insomnia. It helps manage colitis, diverticulosis, flatulence, headaches, pain, and fever. Chamomile is most popularly consumed as a tea or an herbal infusion, and can be consumed regularly without fear of side effects.

Lady's Mantle - This natural medicine has astringent and styptic properties which help in reducing heavy menses and the pain brought on by heavy periods. It helps regulate hormonal levels and acts as an anti-estrogenic herb that regulates cycle timings and relieves cramps. It's also invaluable for women going through menopause since it helps their body adjust to the wild fluctuation of hormonal levels.

Lavender – The infusion of lavender is known to have calming effects which helps reduce stress and fatigue, provides relief from insomnia, and acts as a relaxant and sleep aid. The oil of lavender is also invaluable to calming the nervous system when used as a diffusion or a massage tool.

Lemon Balm – This garden herb is effective in easing discomfort from a myriad of menopause-related conditions: insomnia, fever, headaches, cramps, mild depression, stress, anxiety, palpitations, digestive relaxant during gas, bloating, vomiting, and an upset stomach. It also acts as a cardiotonic and is protective against viral illnesses as well.

Licorice Root – The root of the licorice plant is useful in adjusting and boosting the metabolic processes associated with estrogen, and helps reduce symptoms which are caused by hormone fluctuations. It also acts as an enhancer for the pharmacological action of other herbs, when used in conjunction with them.

Walnut Leaves – These act as an excellent natural remedy and are known to hold astringent, antifungal, antiviral, sedative, and nourishing properties. If used in conjunction with other herbs in an herbal infusion, walnut leaves are highly effective in reducing excessive menstruation.

Shepherd's Purse – This constricts blood vessels and helps reduce blood flow, particularly effective when dealing with heavy bleeding during periods. It is also known to provide strong relief from chronic uterine bleeding disorders, especially due to the presence of uterine fibroids. It is a known remedy for irregular heartbeats, blood pressure problems, nosebleeds, etc. However, caution must be exercised in its use, and you should discuss it with your physician before consumption, especially if you're suffering from blood pressure problems.

Yarrow – It is known to have beneficial effects against problems concerning ovarian function and health, irregular periods, cramps, insomnia, anxiety, stress and menopausal mood swings, etc. It is most effective if used as an infusion or as a tea. It is of such great value as a medicinal herb for female health problems that many herbalists hold it to be one of the most important herbs in existence that provide relief to women.

Chapter   4:   Homeopathic Preparations for Menopause

<u>Arnica</u> **(Arnica montana)** – The homeopathic remedy, Arnica, has long been used as a popular alternative medicine for bruising as well as muscle and joint pain. When used in the form of an herbal rub, topical application of Arnica is extremely effective as a pain reliever, especially to soothe aching muscles and stiff joints.

<u>Lachesis</u> – A homeopathic medicine, Lachesis is well-known as an effective remedy against hot flashes, headaches and migraines.

<u>Sepia</u> – Another effective homeopathic remedy, Sepia has long been used as a natural medicine for relief from menopausal symptoms – depression, indifference, mood swings, vaginal dryness and irritation, as well as pain during intercourse due to lack of lubrication or elasticity.

Chapter 5: Everyday Activities and Alternative Therapies for Menopause

1. Take a 20-minute tepid bath in the morning to reduce hot flashes all day long.

2. Exercising is important to help maintain and regulate blood flow and mood-related problems. Apart from cardio exercises, weight training and other such exercise regimes are recommended to keep bones healthy and sturdy.

3. Anecdotal evidence from countless women, along with research through scientific studies, shows that acupuncture is invaluable in providing relief from most menopausal symptoms when used in conjunction with other alternative herbal remedies, or even without.

4. Reduce consumption of alcohol since it aggravates some symptoms. Also avoid diuretics like coffee and antihistamines since they cause dehydration in the body.

5. Wear natural fiber clothing if pestered with vaginal irritation or infections.

6. A healthy and regular sex life helps keep the vaginal tissues healthy and promotes better blood circulation, natural lubrication, and also uplifts the mood (as long as you're doing it right).

7. Breathing exercises are invaluable in reducing or controlling mood swings and feelings of anxiety and stress brought on by fluctuating hormones.

8. Hypnosis, the therapeutic and licensed kind practiced by medical or psychological professionals, has shown considerable effectiveness in helping women cope with the many symptoms of menopause as well as reducing the magnitude of discomfort from many of them.

9. If you're a smoker, try to quit – since smoking is known to trigger several symptoms such as hot flashes and bladder irritation.

Conclusion

The lack of sufficient research into many of the natural remedies which help treat menopausal symptoms is quite negligent, especially considering that almost 50% of the global population undergoes this completely natural change in their lives. The conclusive evidence regarding the risks of HRT as well as the loud marketing and claims of natural and alternative remedies makes this a confusing and sometimes worrying phase to undergo in the lives of many women.

Many women labor under the wrong impression that "natural" automatically means safe, however, the truth is far from that. Most natural compounds are the starting point for many pharmaceutical products that are prescribed by doctors and sold in pharmacies. The difference is that they aren't as stringently controlled or researched in order to understand their entire range of benefits and adverse side effects. They have just as many strict instructions which need to be followed in terms of dosage, administration, full range and duration of course for maximum benefits, adverse reactions and drug-drug interactions, etc. which many consumers seem to ignore – thinking instead that these natural compounds are a kind of freely consumable candy.

That makes it all the more vital that any alternate therapies and natural remedies that you may be considering be thoroughly discussed and planned in conjunction with your physician. So, after reading this book, highlight a few of the natural therapies you'd like to try, and then discuss them with your doctor.

Finally, I'd like to thank you for buying this book! If you found it helpful, I'd greatly appreciate it if you'd take a moment to leave a review on Amazon. Thank you!

Made in the USA
Las Vegas, NV
20 April 2023

70825713R00024